SIGHT

Wayne Jackman

Reading consultant:
Diana Bentley
University of Reading

Photographs by
Chris Fairclough

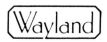

The Senses

Touch
Sight
Hearing
Smell
Taste

Editor: Janet De Saulles

First published in 1989 by
Wayland (Publishers) Ltd
61 Western Road, Hove
East Sussex, BN3 1JD, England

© Copyright 1989 Wayland (Publishers) Ltd

British Library Cataloguing in Publication Data
Jackman, Wayne
　1. Man. Sight
　I. Title II. Series
　612'.84

　　ISBN 1—85210—731—6

Phototypeset by Kalligraphics Ltd, Horley, Surrey, England
Printed and bound by Casterman S.A., Belgium

Contents

All the words that appear
in **bold** are explained in the
glossary on page 22.

Our eyes help us to work and play.

There are five **senses** – sight, touch, smell, hearing and taste. This book is about sight. Look around you at all the things you can see. Can you see the blue sky or a beautiful flower? Maybe you can see a friend. Our sense of sight also helps us. It stops us from bumping into things or having nasty accidents.

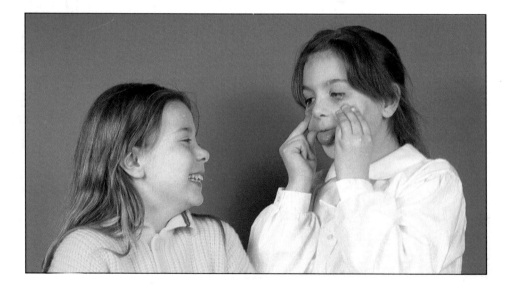

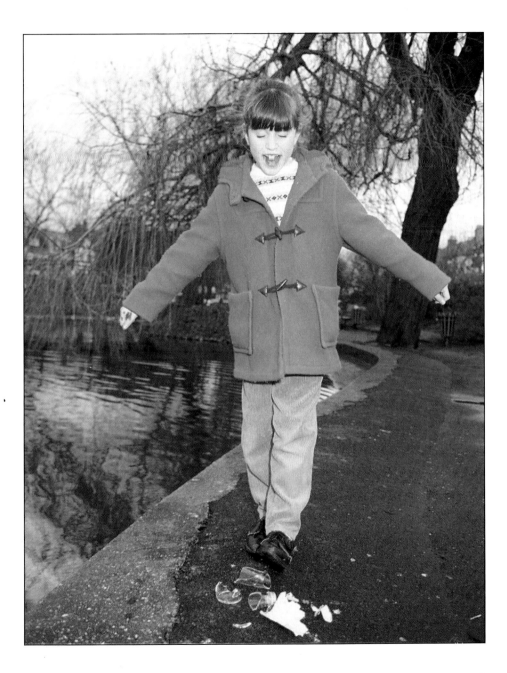

Far and near.

We can see some things easily. This is because they are large or because they are close to us. Other things are very small. So that we can see them better, we look through a **magnifying glass**. Some things are too far away to be seen clearly. We look through a **telescope** to bring them nearer.

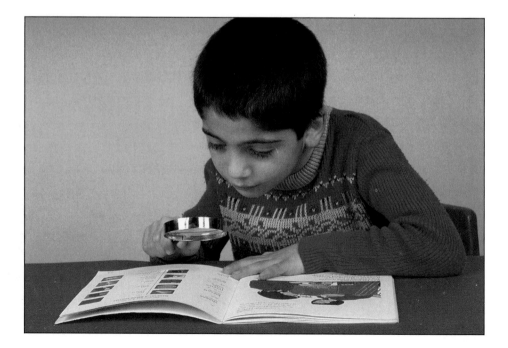

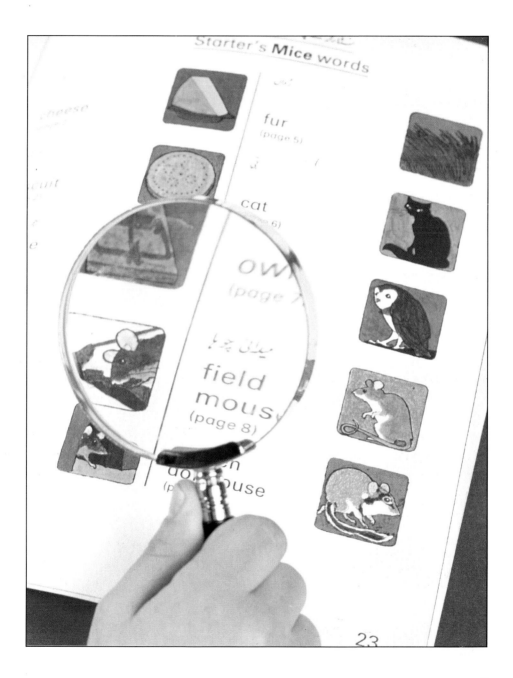

7

I cannot see.

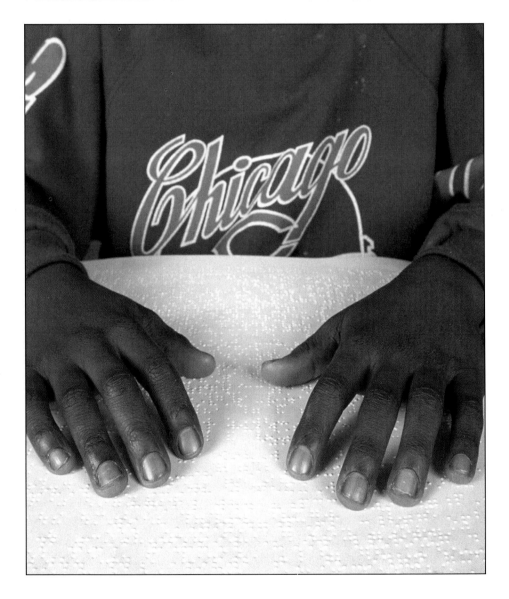

Some people cannot see. They are blind. Imagine what that must be like. Close your eyes and carefully move about. It's difficult! How do blind people read? They use a special system of raised dots called **braille**. Their fingers 'feel' the writing. Find out what this is like. Draw a **maze** and mark the way with a line of pin-pricks. Ask a friend to reach the centre by feeling the holes.

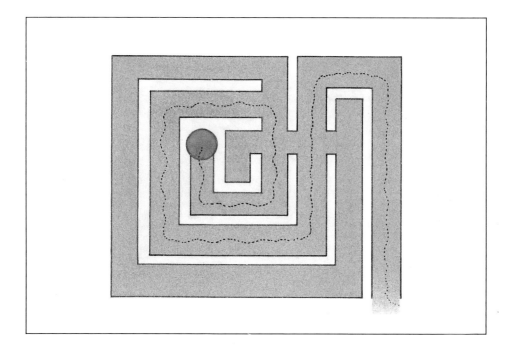

Do you wear glasses?

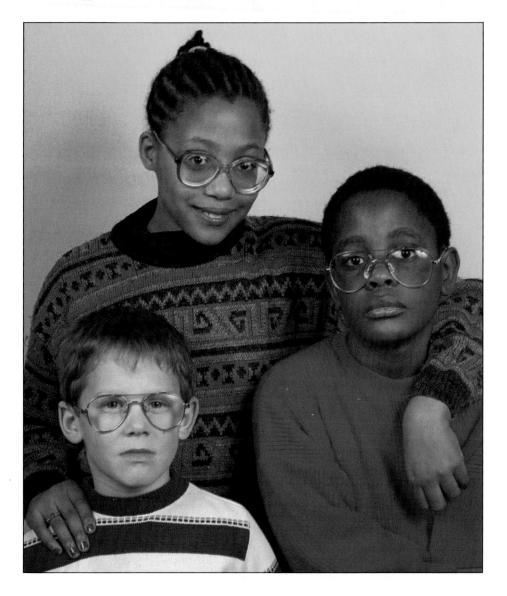

Some people cannot see clearly things which are far away. They are short-sighted. Other people cannot see clearly things which are close. They are long-sighted. To help them see better they wear glasses. Perhaps you do. Now look at the diagram. What can you see? Some people cannot read the number. They are **colour-blind**. They usually think red and green are the same colour.

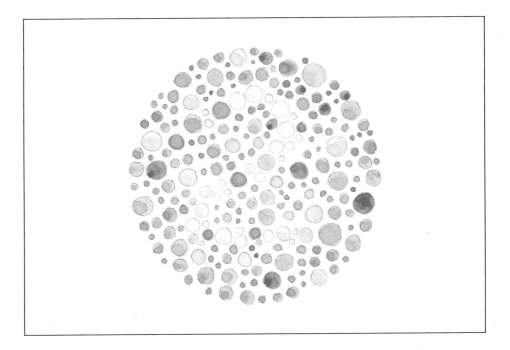

What do our eyes look like?

Our eyes are round and the same size as a ping-pong ball. They see by collecting light. This enters our eyes through the pupil, which is the black dot in the middle of the eye. Around the pupil is the **iris**. This is the coloured part of the eye. What colour are your eyes?

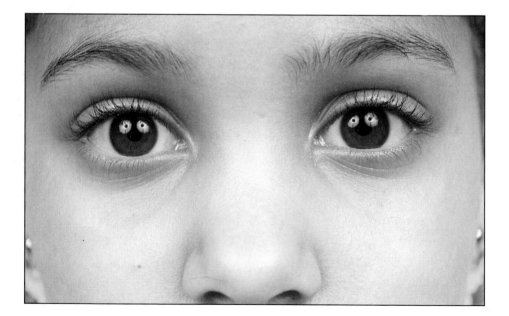

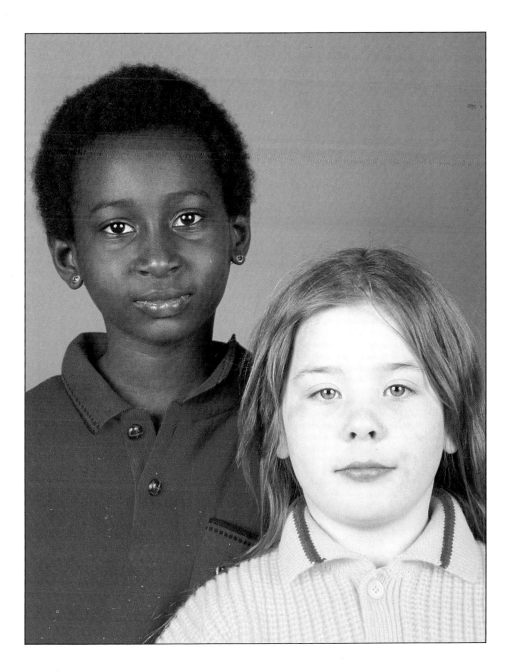

The pupil opens and closes.

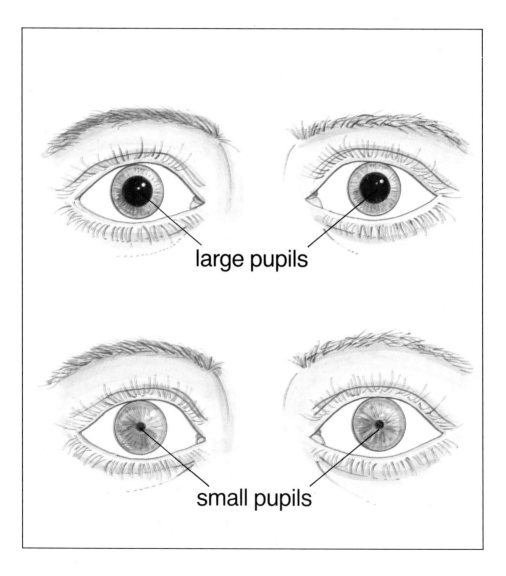

large pupils

small pupils

The pupil is like a tiny window which opens and closes to let in just the right amount of light. Look at the light coming in through a window. Ask a friend if he or she can see your pupils getting smaller. Now shut your eyes for one minute. Can your friend see that your pupils have grown bigger?

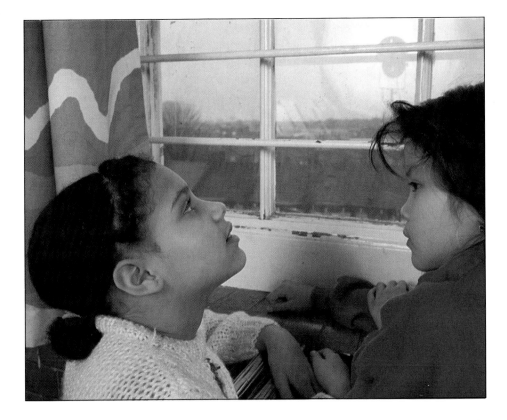

How our eyes are kept clean.

Our eyes are protected from dirt, dust and sweat by our eyebrows and eyelashes. The eyelids are like windscreen wipers. Each time we blink, the eyelids wash salty tears over our eyes. This keeps them clean and moist. Did you know that we blink about thirty times in one minute?

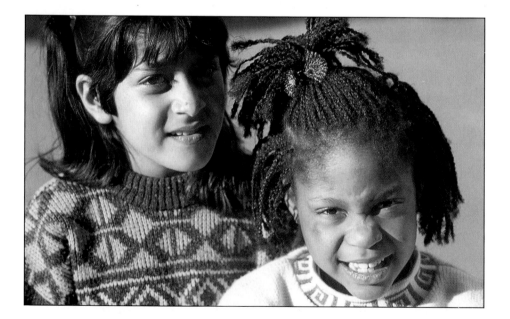

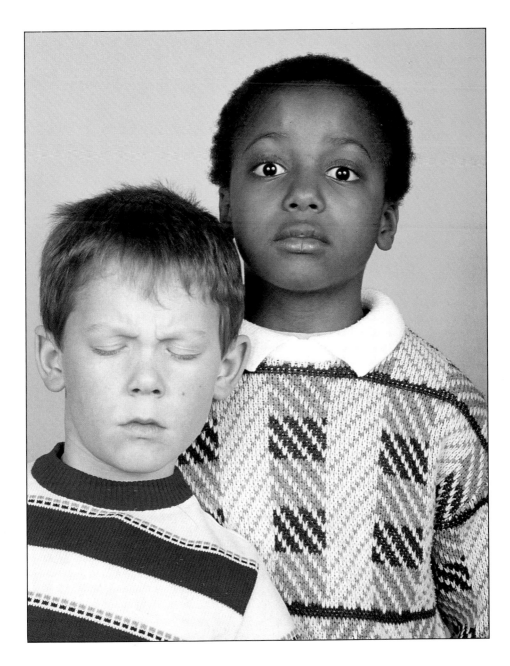

Some games to test our sight.

1. Put your middle fingers together and slowly bring them towards your eyes. What can you see? A string of sausages?

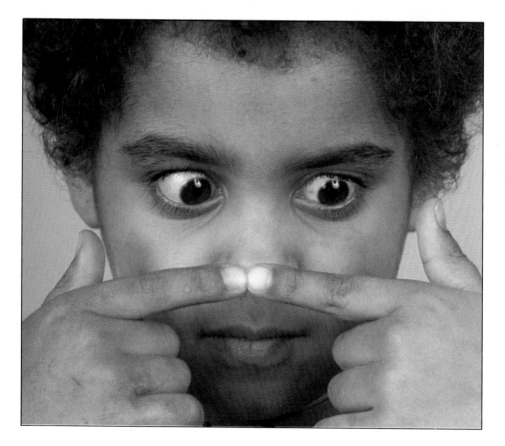

2. With some friends, draw a picture of a rabbit. Pin the picture to the wall. Attach some sticky tape to some cotton wool for the rabbit's tail. Take turns to be blindfolded and stick the tail in place on the rabbit!

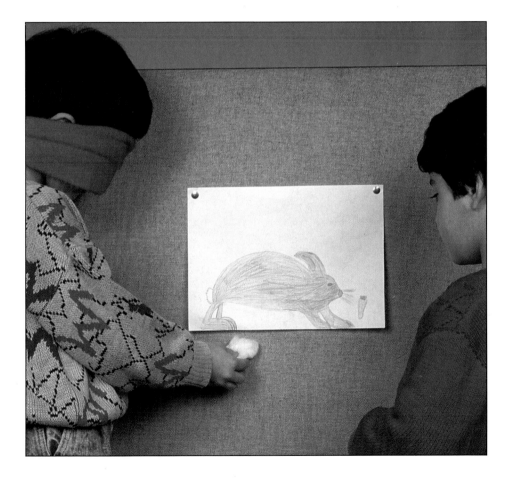

Spots before our eyes.

Our eyes can sometimes play tricks on us. Look at the diagrams below. What can you see?

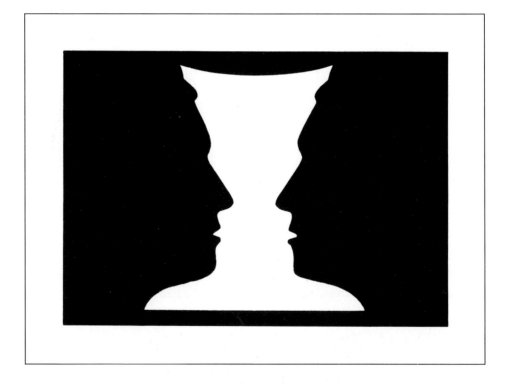

A vase perhaps? Look closely again. Maybe there are two faces.

Judging distances can be difficult. Which line is the longest? Now check with a ruler.

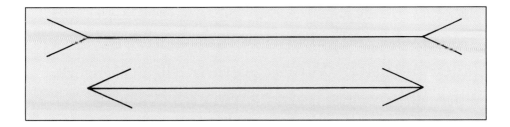

Look at these squares. Wait a second. Now, can you see grey dots where the white lines cross? They aren't really there at all. Look at one of the spots very carefully. Can you see it disappear?

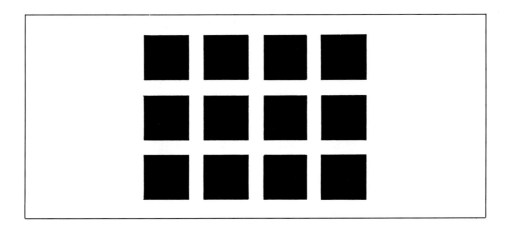

Glossary

Braille A system of writing for the blind. Each letter or number is made up of raised dots which the blind person can feel.

Colour-blind When somebody cannot see the difference between some colours.

Iris The coloured part of the eye which surrounds the pupil.

Magnifying glass This is made of a rounded piece of glass. It makes things look as if they are bigger.

Maze A puzzle where you must find the correct path to the centre.

Senses We use our senses to know what things look, feel, smell, sound and taste like.

Telescope People use one of these in order to see things which are far away. It makes the objects seem nearer.

Books to read

I See With My Eyes by Joan Mills (Schofield & Son, 1986)

Look At Eyes by Ruth Thomson (Franklin Watts, 1988)

Seeing by Henry Pluckrose (Franklin Watts, 1985)

Things I See illustrated by Peter Longden (Ladybird, 1985)

Your Eyes by Joan Iveson-Iveson (Wayland, 1985)

Acknowledgements

The author and the Publisher would like to thank the Headteacher, staff and pupils of Millfield Junior School, Elmcroft Street, London, for their help in producing this book.

23

Index